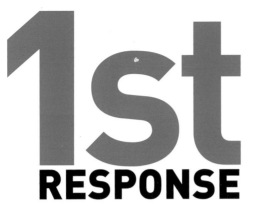

1st
RESPONSE

Participant's course book

To help you manage an
incident with confidence

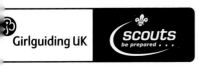

Girlguiding UK scouts be prepared . . .

Girlguiding UK wishes to thank St. John Ambulance, The British Red Cross and The Resuscitation Council (UK) for their help with this publication.

Published in cooperation with The Scout Association by
Girlguiding UK
17-19 Buckingham Palace Road
London SW1W 0PT
Email: chq@girlguiding.org.uk
Website: www.girlguiding.org.uk

ISBN 0 85260 152 2
Girlguiding UK Trading Service ordering code 6525

Printed and bound by Sterling ColourPrint

Working group: Girlguiding UK – Rachel Jacques (Chair) and Heidi Carnall.
The Scout Association – Margaret Medler and Melissa Green
Project Editor: Alison Griffiths
Designer: Angie Daniel
Illustrator: Aces Graphics
Project Coordinator: Danielle Cain, Kaye Hannah

Original 1st Response working group: Sarah Bristow, Judy Morris, Jennie Lamb, Paul Randell, John Cole

Members are reminded that during the lifespan of this publication there may be changes to:
• Girlguiding UK's policy
• The Scout Association's policy
• first aid protocols
which will affect the accuracy of the information contained within these pages.

CONTENTS

Introduction	 5

How to use this book 6
Child protection policy 6

Chapter 1: Principles of first aid	 8

Arrival at an incident 8
Managing an incident 9
Basic life support diagrams 12

Chapter 2: Emergency life support	 14

Primary survey 14
The recovery position 15
Basic life support 16
Life-threatening situations 18
   Shock 18
   Bleeding 19

Chapter 3: The unconscious casualty	 21

Identifying injuries 21
Monitoring the casualty's condition 21
Causes of unconsciousness 22
   Fainting 22
   Imbalance of heat (seizures) 22
   Heart attack 23
   Angina pectoris 23
   Head injuries 23
   Asphyxia/hypoxia 24
      Choking 24
      Near drowning 25
   Asthma 25
   Anaphylactic shock 26
   Poisoning 26
   Seizures 27
   Diabetic emergencies 28
      Hypoglycaemia 28

Chapter 4: Other injuries and conditions · · · · · · · · · · · · · 29

Heat and cold 29
    Heat exhaustion 29
    Heatstroke 29
    Hypothermia 29
    Burns 30
        Chemical burns 30
        Sunburn 31
Fractures and soft tissue injuries 31
    Fractures 31
    Soft tissue injuries (sprains and strains) .32
Minor injuries 32
    Eye injuries 32
    Foreign bodies in the ears and nose 32
    Minor cuts and grazes 32
    Nosebleeds 32
    Tooth loss 33
    Splinters 33
    Stings (and anaphylaxis) 33
    Animal and snake bites 33
Ailments 34
    Tetanus 34
    Meningitis 34
Summary 35

Appendix 1: Infection and the first aider · · · · · · · · · · · · · 36

Appendix 2: First aid kits · · · · · · · · · · · · · 38

Appendix 3: Elevation and arm sling · · · · · · · · · · · · · 40

Appendix 4: Chain of survival · · · · · · · · · · · · · 41

Appendix 5: Further resources · · · · · · · · · · · · · 42

Appendix 6: Useful addresses · · · · · · · · · · · · · 43

INTRODUCTION

Welcome to this revised edition of the *1st Response Participant's course book*, which has been fully updated to include current resuscitation guidelines. The book contains simple first aid information that is relevant to Leaders within Girlguiding UK and The Scout Association. It can be used on its own or with an up-to-date first aid manual.

The 1st Response course is designed to help Guiding and Scouting Leaders to build confidence and skills in coping with first aid emergency situations – at the meeting place, out and about on activities or at residential events. The 1st Response training will equip you with the knowledge needed to manage these emergencies. You will need to remain calm for the sake of the young people present and use other adults to assist you until more experienced help arrives. You will be required to keep your skills updated by attending regular trainings.

It is important that you get to know about any medical conditions relevant to the young people in your care and other adult helpers. If a particular condition is not covered by 1st Response, find out as much as you can about it: talk to parents/ guardians or the adult helper, seek advice from the relevant Association Adviser in your area, and contact specialist organisations for more information. If you are well informed you will be in a good position to help if an emergency situation should occur.

The *1st Response Participant's course book* does not cover risk assessment, your Association's relevant child protection policy or personal hygiene. You will need to refer to your organisation's resources for information on these subjects (see Further resources, page 42).

We wish you well in all your activities and hope they are accident-free!

Chair, 1st Response Working Group

HOW TO USE THIS BOOK

Members of Girlguiding UK and The Scout Association have prepared this course book for your use as part of a basic course on first aid and incident management. The book contains information about first aid, but is by no means a first aid manual. At the 1st Response training you will learn the skills outlined in this book, though the course does not replace a full assessed first aid course. If you want to learn more, see pages 43–44 for details of organisations that can offer further resources and training.

This course covers the requirements of Girlguiding UK's and The Scout Association's leadership schemes. Your skills should be refreshed at least every three years, in line with all other first aid certificates.

The course is designed to last one day, or two evenings. This includes time to practise the skills you learn as well as time for discussion and exercises to reinforce your learning.

CHILD PROTECTION POLICY

Both Girlguiding UK and The Scout Association have compiled their own child protection policies and you must be familiar with the relevant policy (see Further resources, page 42). First aid involves necessary handling of casualties and though having a second person present is ideal, it is not always possible in an emergency situation. Always explain to the casualty what you are doing, regardless of their level of consciousness.

For all procedures in this book it is assumed that the first aider is not alone with the casualty, so that there is someone else present to call for help.

DUTY OF CARE FOR OTHER PEOPLE'S CHILDREN

While first aiders would not normally give medication, youth leaders working with other people's children have a duty of care equivalent to that of a 'responsible parent'. They are often required to care for or carry medicines for young children, and sometimes need to administer them.

Leaders in Guiding and Scouting may give medication with a parent's prior permission in these circumstances:

- Parents/guardians supply medication for the unit meeting/holiday/camp/trip for an immediate condition, eg antibiotics, travel pills or for an expected problem like hay fever or migraines.

- Parents/guardians supply medication for the unit meeting/holiday/camp/trip for a known medical condition, such as asthma or diabetes. Medicines, including for example inhalers and Epipens, will need to be taken as prescribed. Some of the conditions listed above are covered in the 1st Response course. For further help, Guiders and Scouters are encouraged to seek help and/or training from parents, County Advisers or appropriate organisations such as Diabetes UK.

Commonly used medication for minor illnesses such as a sore throat, virus or flu-like symptoms may be carried by the first aider; for example, paracetamol, throat lozenges, insect bite and sting relief. Prior to residential events, parents/guardians should be asked on the appropriate form to give permission for the Leader to use this medication at their discretion. Girlguiding UK members record this on the General Health Form. Members of The Scout Association should see *First Aid Kits and Accident Books* (FS140048) for further guidance.

If a child becomes ill during an event or trip and the Leaders feel that it would be appropriate to give medication which they do not already have permission to give, they should contact the parent/guardian by phone to seek permission. If a Leader is unable to make contact, the Leader will be authorised by the Children Act to take reasonable steps to safeguard a child, which extend to administering appropriate medication if common sense suggests it is needed.

Administering medication
Prior to giving any medication, Leaders must check expiry dates and give the correct dose at the correct time. These details must be recorded.

1 PRINCIPLES OF FIRST AID

There are three basic principles of first aid:
1 Preserve life - by using simple life-preserving skills, based on the AB of resuscitation: Airway, Breathing (see pages 14–15).
2 Prevent deterioration - by treating life-threatening conditions such as bleeding and shock.
3 Promote recovery - by reassuring the casualty, putting her in an appropriate position and protecting her from the elements and other dangers.

First aid is just that – the help administered by the first person at the scene of an incident. It is not complicated, nor does it require a great deal of equipment.

ARRIVAL AT AN INCIDENT

The first person arriving at an incident should know what to do so that valuable time is not lost:

1 Check your safety.
2 Make safe.
3 Give emergency aid.
4 Get help.

Do not rush into a situation until you are sure that it is safe to approach. You cannot afford to get injured – if you do, who will help? Be aware of hidden dangers:
- People who may make a situation worse.
- Objects that could get in the way or jeopardise safety.
- Electricity, gas or fumes. Protect yourself by turning off the mains, ventilating the room etc.
- Spilled fluids.
- Fire.
- Dangerous buildings.
- Environmental dangers such as unstable rocks, rising tide.
- Other traffic at a road traffic accident – get someone to control it. If applicable, put on the car's handbrake, switch off the engine and check for spilled petrol.

It is important to get as much information as possible so that you can assess a situation.
- Look around the scene of the incident.
- If possible, ask the casualty questions, for example whether and

8

where she feels pain (symptoms). Listen to what the casualty tells you; even a small child will know what is painful and what 'feels right' and will be able to indicate her wishes.

- Ask bystanders what happened (history).
- Check for any obvious injuries. Always explain to the casualty what you are doing.
- Look for any medical bracelets or medicines on the casualty.

Bear in mind that in looking for medical bracelets etc your actions may be misinterpreted. Explain to the casualty and those around why you are taking these actions.

MANAGING AN INCIDENT
Do not exceed your capabilities
Keep your treatment simple and do what is necessary. Do not try to exceed your capabilities and always send for help if it is needed.

Prioritise
Check how many casualties there are. Think about who needs help most urgently.

- Noisy casualties have open airways and should not necessarily be looked at first.
- Get bystanders to help, bearing in mind the rest of your group and child protection issues.
- If someone with more knowledge arrives, let her take over – you can assist as requested.

Get help
This may involve sending someone to telephone for the emergency services or letting a parent/guardian know that a minor incident (eg grazed knee) has taken place.

In a serious emergency, it is important to get help as quickly as possible. Get someone you can trust to go to a telephone. Make sure she has a clear message to give, including:

- the number of casualties and a description of their conditions: whether conscious or unconscious and whether breathing or not
- where you are, including any landmarks and your postcode
- what sort of help is needed.

Ask the person to return and confirm that this has been done.

It is important to remember that any incident can be traumatic for bystanders and especially children. Where possible, use another member of your group to take children away from the scene. Be sure to debrief the incident with all involved at the earliest opportunity.

Report the incident
Both Girlguiding UK and The Scout Association have rules about reporting an incident.

- Girlguiding UK requires the casualty's parent/guardian and the appropriate Commissioner to be informed and a Notification of Accident or Incident form (available at www.girlguiding.org.uk) to be filled in and returned to the insurance provider. See Useful addresses (page 43).

- The Scout Association requires a leader to report all incidents to the casualty's parent/guardian. In cases where the casualty has required or could require medical aid, ie from a hospital or doctor, the Scout Information Centre (0845 300 1818) will need to be informed. Accidents that are serious, life threatening or fatal need to be reported to the Public Relations team (0845 300 1818).

Check the incident reporting procedure before an event. Reports should state:

- the time and date (including the year) of the incident
- what happened
- who was involved
- what action was taken
- whether there were witnesses.

If in doubt contact your Commissioner for up-to-date information.

First aid equipment

Although first aid is generally performed with little or no equipment, good practice with any first aid kit includes:

- equipping it according to the size of the event and age of the participants
- not keeping any medication or ointments in the kit (these should be kept separately according to different storage needs)
- not keeping unnecessary equipment
- not overstocking – products can go out of date or get damaged

- replacing items as they are used. See Appendix 2 (page 38) for a guide to first aid kit contents.

Protect yourself from infection

There is always a small risk that you might pick up an infection when undertaking first aid. Always try to wear disposable gloves when undertaking first aid. Try to make a habit of carrying gloves. If gloves are not available, improvise with polythene bags. It is also useful to carry a face shield. After treatment, remove and dispose of the gloves/shield carefully and wash your hands thoroughly with soap and water. Contaminated surfaces etc should be washed with bleach diluted with 1:10 parts water. If you are worried that you may have been exposed to infection, contact your GP or local accident and emergency unit as soon as possible.

Your trainer may show you a face shield which is placed over the casualty's face during mouth-to-mouth ventilations.

See Appendix 1 (page 36) for more information.

EMERGENCY LIFE SUPPORT FOR ADULTS AND CHILDREN

Primary survey

CHECK FOR DANGER.

1 CHECK FOR RESPONSE. ▶
SPEAK LOUDLY AND CLEARLY TO THE CASUALTY. ASK QUESTIONS LIKE 'ARE YOU ALL RIGHT?'.

IF THERE IS NO RESPONSE, SHOUT FOR HELP. DO NOT LEAVE THE CASUALTY.

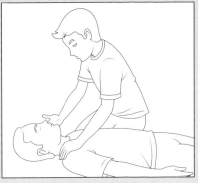

2 OPEN THE AIRWAY. ▼

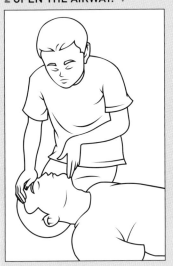

3 CHECK FOR NORMAL BREATHING. LOOK, LISTEN AND FEEL. ▼

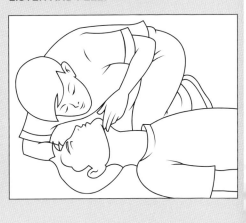

4 IF BREATHING NORMALLY, PLACE IN THE RECOVERY POSITION. ▼

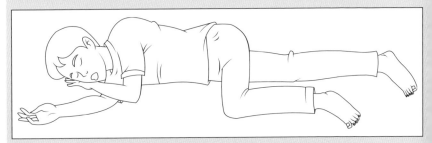

CALL THE EMERGENCY SERVICES.

EMERGENCY LIFE SUPPORT FOR ADULTS AND CHILDREN

Basic life support

CARRY OUT A PRIMARY SURVEY:
- **DANGER**
- **RESPONSE**
- **AIRWAY**
- **BREATHING**

CALL THE EMERGENCY SERVICES.

FOR CHILDREN
IT CAN BE MORE BENEFICIAL TO GIVE FIVE INITIAL RESCUE BREATHS FOLLOWED BY CYCLES OF 30:2 COMPRESSIONS AND BREATHS. ONE-HANDED COMPRESSIONS MAY BE MORE SUITABLE.

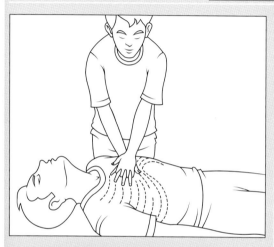

1 IF NOT BREATHING NORMALLY, START CPR WITH 30 CHEST COMPRESSIONS. ▲

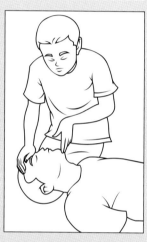

2 OPEN THE AIRWAY. ▲

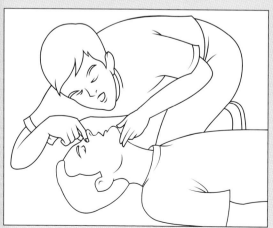

3 GIVE TWO RESCUE BREATHS. ◄

CONTINUE WITH 30 COMPRESSIONS AND TWO RESCUE BREATHS UNTIL:
- QUALIFIED HELP ARRIVES TO TAKE OVER
- THE CASUALTY STARTS TO BREATHE NORMALLY
- YOU BECOME TOO EXHAUSTED TO CONTINUE.

2 EMERGENCY LIFE SUPPORT

PRIMARY SURVEY

In the previous chapter it was stressed that the first principle of first aid is to preserve life. This is done by following the mnemonic **DRAB**:

D – **D**anger
R – **R**esponse
A – **A**irway
B – **B**reathing

Check for danger

- Check that it is safe to approach the casualty.
- Do not move the casualty unless he is in danger.

Check for response

Establish whether or not the casualty is conscious:

- Speak loudly and clearly to the casualty. Ask questions like 'Are you all right?', 'What's your name?', 'Can you open your eyes?'.
- If there is no response, gently shake the casualty's shoulders and ask loudly 'Are you all right?'.
- If there is a coherent response, find out what is wrong and deal with the situation.
- If there is no response, shout out for help. Do not leave the casualty.

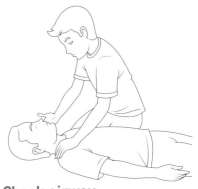

Check airway

An unconscious casualty's airway may be blocked or restricted, making breathing difficult or impossible.

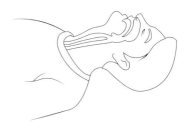

- Open the airway by placing one hand on his forehead and tilting the head back gently. Place two fingers beneath the chin on the jaw bone and gently lift the chin upwards and forwards.

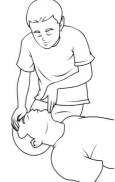

Check breathing

Kneel beside the casualty. Supporting his chin with the airway open, place your cheek close to his mouth and nose:

- **Look –** down the chest and abdomen for breathing movements.
- **Listen –** for sounds of breathing.
- **Feel –** for warm breath on your face.
- Do this for ten seconds.
- If the casualty is not breathing normally, proceed to resuscitation (page 16).
- If he is breathing normally, place him in the recovery position.

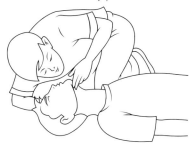

THE RECOVERY POSITION FOR ADULTS AND CHILDREN

Any unconscious, breathing casualty should be placed in the recovery position. This ensures that he is supported on his side with the airway open, allowing secretions to drain out.

What to do:

1 Kneel beside the casualty.

2 Remove spectacles (if applicable) and check the casualty's pockets.

3 If necessary, gently straighten the legs.

4 Place the nearest arm to you at right angles to the body with the elbow bent (do not force it) and the palm facing upwards.

5▶ Bring the far arm across the chest, placing your palm in the casualty's palm, with the back of the casualty's hand against the cheek.

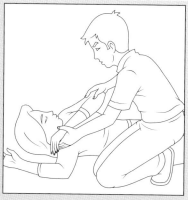

◀6 Using your other hand, grab the far leg at the knee and pull it up, ensuring the foot remains on the ground.

7 Keeping the palm of your hand against the side of the casualty's face so that you are supporting the airway, pull the far knee and gently roll the casualty towards you until lying on one side.

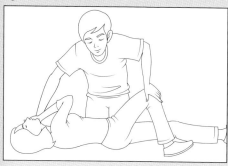

▶▶

8 Tilt the head gently to ensure that the airway is open. Adjust the hand under the cheek if necessary to achieve this.

▼**9** Adjust the upper leg so that the hip and knee are at right angles.

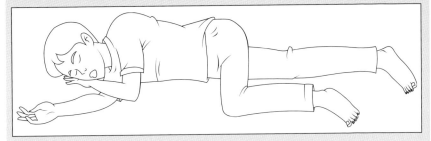

10 Check the casualty's breathing and monitor frequently.

11 Cover the casualty with a blanket if available.

Once the casualty is in the recovery position he can be left safely while you get help, if it has not already been sent for. On returning, monitor his condition and regularly check his breathing.

A casualty should be moved gently into the recovery position from any position he may have been found in, unless the airway is already open and the casualty stable.

BASIC LIFE SUPPORT

Cardiopulmonary resuscitation (CPR) is unlikely to bring a casualty 'back to life' but it can prevent damage to vital organs, thereby giving a casualty a 'fighting chance'. Therefore, it is important to continue CPR until the emergency services arrive.

The following technique is suitable for use on adult and child casualties. See page 18 for additional notes on basic life support for children.

What to do:

Do a primary survey (DRAB). If a casualty is not breathing normally or has agonal breathing (see note opposite):

1 Send someone you trust to call for an ambulance and ask him to come back and tell you he has done it. If you are on your own you will need to do this.

2 Kneel by the casualty.

3 Grasping your hands together, place the heel of your hand in the centre of the casualty's chest. ▶▶

4▶ Interlock the fingers of your hands and position yourself vertically above the casualty's chest. With your arms straight, press down onto the sternum (breast bone) to a depth of about 4–5cm.

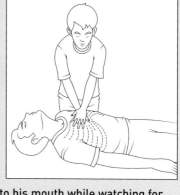

5 After each compression, release all pressure on the sternum without losing contact. Repeat 30 times. Do not apply any pressure over the ribs or upper abdomen.

▼6 After 30 compressions, open the casualty's airway using the head tilt and chin lift. Pinch the nose and make a good seal around the casualty's mouth. Blow steadily into his mouth while watching for the chest to rise. If the chest does not rise, re-check that the head is in the

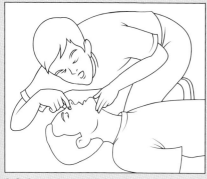

correct position. Make sure that you have a good seal around the mouth. Look to see whether there is any obstruction in the mouth (do not use your fingers to check for obstructions). Now do one more rescue breath.

7 Continue with the compressions and rescue breaths at a ratio of 30:2 and a rate of 100 chest compressions per minute (a little less than two compressions a second).

8 Only stop to recheck the casualty if he starts breathing normally.

If more than one person is present, take turns performing CPR to prevent fatigue.

Continue CPR until:
● qualified help arrives to take over
● the casualty starts to breathe normally
● you become too exhausted.

Agonal breathing is short, infrequent gasps. It is seen in the first few minutes after the heart has stopped.

Chest compression only CPR

If you are unwilling or not able to give rescue breaths, give chest compressions only at a rate of 100 a minute.

- If the casualty starts breathing, turn him into the recovery position (see pages 15–16) and monitor.

Defibrillation

Public Access Defibrillators (PADs) are becoming more accessible, for example in shopping centres, entertainment venues and public areas. If available, telephone instructions may be given by the ambulance service. The operator will ask if a defibrillator is available and give instructions. Once opened, the defibrillator itself will also give instructions.

You may want to obtain defibrillator training at a future date.

CPR is a skill which must be taught by a trained person and practised only on a resuscitation manikin.

Basic life support for children

A 'child' usually refers to someone between the ages of one and puberty. You can perform CPR on a child as you would for an adult, although these additional steps are considered more beneficial.

- Begin with five rescue breaths before starting cycles of 30:2 compressions to breaths.

- If you are alone with a child, do one minute of CPR before going for help.
- When doing chest compressions on a child, compress to one third of the depth of the chest, using one hand.

LIFE-THREATENING SITUATIONS

To prevent deterioration of a casualty's condition, you need to consider conditions that may become life-threatening, eg shock and bleeding.

Shock

Shock is a serious condition caused by both illness and injuries.

The principal causes are:
- bleeding and fluid loss (shock may be the only symptom of internal bleeding)
- the heart's inability to pump sufficient blood around the body (for example in a heart attack)
- an allergic reaction (anaphylaxis).

These conditions result in insufficient oxygen being available to the vital organs (the brain, heart, lungs and kidneys). The body attempts to put this right by drawing blood away from other parts of the body, such as the extremities and the less important organs.

Symptoms of shock:
- The casualty's skin becomes pale and clammy.
- He feels cold, dry-mouthed and nauseous (sick).
- His pulse and breathing rates increase.
- He may become anxious, confused or irrational.
- His level of consciousness may drop.

What to do:

In most first aid situations, shock can be minimised by:
1 Reassuring the casualty.
2 Laying him down (see note below).
3 Raising his legs.
4 Loosening tight clothing.
5 Keeping him warm with a blanket.
6 As far as possible, treating the cause of the shock.

It is important not to give the casualty anything to eat or drink. You may moisten his lips if necessary.

If the casualty is thought to be having a heart attack or has breathing difficulties or chest injuries, he should ideally be supported in a half sitting ('W') position with the knees slightly bent and supported (see page 23).

Bleeding

If a casualty is bleeding, prompt action is required to reduce blood loss and the effects of shock.

What to do:

1 Apply direct pressure to the wound.
2 If possible, elevate the affected area – this encourages the clotting process by restricting the blood flow to the wound.
3▼ Apply a dressing and hold it in place with a bandage. Apply one additional dressing on top of the first if the blood comes through. If it continues to come through remove all dressings and apply new ones.

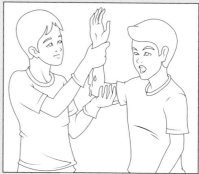

4 Check that bandages on the limbs are not too tight by feeling the area below the bandage (the extremities). If this area is cold or blue, loosen the bandage slightly.

Foreign bodies in wounds

If there is a foreign body in the wound, such as glass:
- Apply pressure above and below the wound.
- Never attempt to remove any foreign body as it might be helping to stem the loss of blood.

Internal bleeding

Internal bleeding can be difficult to identify. A casualty who is bleeding internally may have either a history of injury or a medical condition. You may be able to identify internal bleeding by:

- external signs of injury, such as bruising
- signs of bleeding from an orifice (eg ears, mouth, nose)
- recognising symptoms of shock, which may be the only sign of internal bleeding.

What to do:

1 Place the casualty in the most comfortable position – the recovery position if he is unconscious (see pages 15–16) – and treat for shock.
2 Get him to hospital as soon as possible. Do not waste time trying to identify the cause or attempting to treat it.

3 THE UNCONSCIOUS CASUALTY

Anyone in your care who has been unconscious or less than alert (see page 22) should be checked at a hospital, even if she appears to be recovering well. Never take any risks with those in your care. Anyone who is unconscious must be carefully placed in the recovery position (see pages 15–16) and her breathing, signs of circulation (including facial colour, warmth and movement) monitored, since levels of consciousness can change rapidly. Keep the casualty warm.

Give all the details of the care to whoever takes over her care.

IDENTIFYING INJURIES

Find out what has happened by:
- looking around at the scene of the incident
- asking what happened
- asking the casualty a series of questions, eg 'Do you feel sick?', 'Can you breathe?', 'Are you in any pain?', 'Do you feel dizzy?'.
- looking for signs of injury or illness
- looking for any medical information on the casualty, eg bracelet, card or medication
- briefly checking the body for any injuries.

Always explain to the casualty what you are doing, regardless of her level of consciousness.

MONITORING THE CASUALTY'S CONDITION

It is very important to monitor a casualty's condition constantly, particularly if she is unconscious. The information you pass on may be crucial. The signs you should look for are:
- an open airway
- breathing
- any physical change in her condition – eg colour (if there is insufficient contrast because of skin tone, check inside her lips), temperature etc
- any change of consciousness, eg her response level.

If possible, write your observations down and pass the information on to the person who takes over from you. Any relevant evidence (such as poisons found etc) must be kept and given to medical personnel.

Remember that an unconscious casualty may be aware of you, so constantly reassure her. It is important to establish whether or not the casualty is able to respond to you.

There are four levels of consciousness, which can be remembered as **AVPU**:

....

A – **A**lert – will talk but may be drowsy.

V – Responds to **V**oice – responds to simple commands, eg 'Open your eyes', or may respond to simple questions.

P – Responds to **P**ain – will react (eg make a noise) to a pinch on the back of her hand.

U – **U**nresponsive – there is no response at all.

....

CAUSES OF UNCONSCIOUSNESS

There are a number of causes of unconsciousness. The principal causes are:

● fainting
● imbalance of heat (seizures)
● shock
● heart attack/angina pectoris
● head injuries
● asphyxia/hypoxia/drowning/choking
● asthma
● anaphylactic shock
● poisoning
● seizures
● diabetic emergencies.

Fainting

Fainting can occur for a number of reasons. These include:

● reaction to pain, fright or upset
● exhaustion, lack of food or fluid
● becoming too hot or too cold
● being unwell.

Fainting is caused by a temporary reduction in blood flow to the brain, leading to a brief loss of consciousness.

What to do:

1 Lay the casualty down, raise her legs and loosen tight clothing.
2 Reassure her as she recovers and gradually sit her up.
3 If she does not start to regain consciousness, put her in the recovery position (see pages 15–16) and get help.
4 Check for any injuries in the case of a fall.
5 Try to find the cause of the faint.

Imbalance of heat (seizures)

This type of seizure is usually only seen in children under the age of three. Seizures are caused by a rapid increase in body temperature due to an infection.

What to do:

1 Seek urgent medical advice. Position soft padding around the casualty so that she is protected from injuries caused by violent movements.
2 Remove clothing as far as possible, but be careful not to overcool her.
3 Cool her down by fanning or sponging her with tepid water.
4 Once the movement has stopped, place the casualty in the recovery position to keep the airway open and continue to monitor her condition, especially her breathing.

Often liquid paracetamol is administered before (if previous history is known) or shortly afterwards on medical advice – if parental permission has been given.

Shock
See page 18.

Heart attack
The heart is a muscular organ that circulates blood around the body and to the lungs. Heart attacks are often caused by an obstruction to the blood supply to part of the heart muscle, such as a blood clot in a coronary artery.

Before a heart attack the casualty may complain of feeling unwell and may experience indigestion-like pain. During an attack she may:
- experience severe crushing central chest pain which may radiate down her left arm or up her neck
- become very short of breath
- look ashen in colour and her lips and fingers may become blue
- experience sudden faintness or dizziness
- have a rapid, weak or irregular pulse
- have a sense of impending doom
- suddenly collapse.

What to do:
1 If she is still conscious, sit her up, supporting her from behind with her knees slightly bent (the 'W' position).

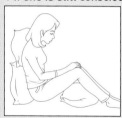

2 Send for urgent medical help.
3 Monitor her carefully. If she has any medication for angina, encourage her to take it. Constantly monitor her level of response, circulation and breathing until help arrives.
4 If she loses consciousness, put her in the recovery position (see pages 15–16) if still breathing normally.
5 If breathing deteriorates, begin CPR (see page 16).

If the casualty is thought to be having a heart attack, or has breathing difficulties or chest injuries, she should ideally be supported in the half sitting ('W') position (see diagram).

Angina pectoris
The coronary arteries supply oxygen to the heart. With age, these arteries become less elastic and tend to narrow. This can lead to a condition called angina pectoris, which causes chest pain and shortness of breath. This can be controlled with medication.

What to do:
1 Help the casualty to sit down.
2 Help her to take her own medication (if available).
3 Encourage her to rest.
4 If the pain persists or returns, seek urgent medical help.

Head injuries
Head injuries can be very serious. For this reason the casualty's parent/guardian or person she lives with must be informed of even an apparently minor bump to the head, since symptoms can be delayed. All head injuries must be taken seriously.

What to do:

1 Treat the casualty with care.

2 Monitor her carefully for nausea, sickness, headache, dizziness or visual problems.

3 If she falls below the 'alert' level of consciousness (see AVPU, page 22), call an ambulance and get her to hospital immediately.

4 If there are signs of any discharge from her eyes, ears or nose, place her in a position to allow this to flow out. Reassure her and get urgent medical help.

5 If the casualty has any symptoms, take her to hospital for a check-up. If in any doubt call NHS Direct for advice: 0845 4647.

Asphyxia/hypoxia

These conditions are caused when insufficient oxygen reaches the body tissues from the blood, as a result of suffocation, choking, near drowning, hanging, strangling or inhalation of fumes. The casualty will experience rapid and/or distressed breathing and gasping. If not treated this will result in restlessness, headache, nausea or vomiting, difficulty in speaking, confusion and unconsciousness. The casualty may stop breathing.

Treat the casualty by, if possible, removing or relieving the cause (see below) and monitoring her condition. If you are worried, get help.

Choking

What to do:

For adults or children over the age of one year who remain conscious:

1 If there is a mild obstruction and the casualty can speak, encourage her to cough.

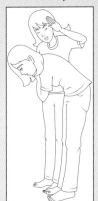

2◀ If there is a severe airway obstruction (casualty is unable to speak) give five back blows. Supporting the chest with one hand, lean the casualty forward and give five sharp blows between the shoulder blades with the heel of the other hand.

3▼ Check to see if the airway obstruction has been relieved. If not, give up to five abdominal thrusts. Stand behind the casualty and put both arms round the upper part of the abdomen. Lean the casualty forward. Clench your fist and place at the bottom of the breast bone. With your other hand, grasp around the fist and pull sharply inwards and upwards.

4 Continue with five back blows and five abdominal thrusts. If the airway is not cleared after three cycles, call the emergency services.

If the casualty becomes unconscious, start CPR.

These techniques should not be practised on a person who is not choking.

Near drowning

If a person is drowning the first thing you may think of is jumping into the water to save her. This, however, may endanger you as well as the casualty.

What to do:
1 Choose the safest way to get the casualty out of the water. Stay on land and try to reach her with your hand or use a stick or rope to pull her in.
2 If the casualty is unconscious you may choose to go into the water. Only do so if you are certain of your own safety. Wading is safer than swimming.
3 Lay the casualty down on a coat or blanket.
4 Check her breathing and commence CPR (with five initial rescue breaths) if she is not breathing normally (see pages 15–17).
5 Treat the casualty for hypothermia (see page 29). Replace her wet clothing and protect her from cold.
6 Take or send her to hospital, even if she appears to have recovered.

Asthma

Asthma is a very variable, allergic condition of the airways; it is very common in children. The symptoms of asthma are wheezing, coughing (especially at night), tightness of the chest and breathlessness. Asthma symptoms may be triggered by exposure to many factors. Some common allergens that are very relevant to Guiding and Scouting include:
- house dust mites
- tree or flower pollens
- pets, especially long-haired animals
- exposure to extreme temperatures
- exercise
- fatigue/tiredness
- medicines, for example paracetamol.

It is very important that the person is aware of her own triggers, especially prior to an event, camp or holiday, so that preventive measures can be taken in advance. You need to discuss with the member and/or parents the signs, symptoms, medication and aftercare of this condition.

It is important that the asthma sufferer has her reliever inhaler (usually blue) with her at all times.

What to do:
1 Keep calm. Allow the casualty to use her reliever inhaler: up to ten individual puffs, via an aerochamber or volumatic spacer device if available. (If not, a paper cup with a hole cut in it can be used.)
2 Allow the person to find a comfortable position, usually sitting up and leaning forward, in a well-ventilated room. Avoid extremes of room temperature.
3 If the person is not responding to the reliever inhaler after five minutes, call the emergency services. Continue to use the reliever inhaler while waiting for the ambulance to arrive.
4 Monitor the airway, breathing and circulation at all times.

For more information contact Asthma UK (see page 43).

Anaphylactic shock

This is a life-threatening reaction that affects the whole body following contact with a trigger. It is very important that the person avoids contact with known triggers. The most common triggers are:

- food products including nuts, fish, dairy produce, soft fruit
- exposure to latex materials ie balloons, rubbers, gloves
- insect bites and stings.

Signs and symptoms develop very quickly following exposure to the trigger. They include:

- tingling of the lips
- swelling of the mouth and lips
- rash starting on the face and spreading over the body
- nausea and vomiting
- abdominal pain
- acute bronchospasm wheezing
- dizziness, collapse and unconsciousness.

What to do:

If a person is aware that she suffers from anaphylactic shock, she may carry adrenaline in the form of a pre-loaded auto injector known as an Epipen or Anapen. In order to administer this you will need to receive training from an appropriate person and parental consent.

The Epipen/Anapen is prescribed by the person's doctor. It should be labelled with the person's name and an expiry date, which must be checked prior to use. It should be administered into the outer thigh, midway between the knee and hip joint (it can be done through clothing).

It is important to discuss with parents and/or members the signs, symptoms, medication and aftercare of this condition.

1 Call the emergency services.
2 When you have done this, immediately administer adrenaline via the Epipen/Anapen.
3 Treat the person for shock. If conscious, use the sitting position (page 23); if unconscious, use the recovery position (pages 15–16). Monitor her airway, breathing and circulation at all times. Do not leave the casualty.
4 Ask another adult to contact the casualty's parents or guardians and keep them updated regarding treatment and hospital treatment.

A second Epipen/Anapen may be needed after 15 minutes if the patient's condition has not improved and the ambulance has not arrived, and the casualty has a second Epipen/Anapen with her.

For more information contact The Anaphylaxis Campaign (see page 43).

Poisoning

Poisons are substances that are toxic to the body. They can include alcohol, drugs and misused substances. Poisons can be inhaled, swallowed, absorbed through the skin or injected. They cause temporary or permanent damage to the body. Any poison that has entered the body will continue to do damage until the body has removed it naturally or treatment has been given. Poisoning requires urgent medical treatment.

What to do:

1 If possible, try to identify what the poison was by asking the casualty or looking for empty containers etc.
2 Call an ambulance and give as much information about what has been swallowed as possible. Alternatively, seek advice from NHS Direct: 0845 4647.
3 Swallowed poisons can burn the lips, mouth and food passages. Never induce vomiting in anyone who has swallowed poison. See also Chemical burns (page 30).
4 If the casualty's lips are burnt, give her sips, never more than this, of cold water (or milk in the case of corrosive poisons) to help prevent swelling, while waiting for help to arrive.
5 If the casualty does vomit, retain it and send it to the hospital with her.
6 Get her to hospital immediately.

Seizures (epileptic and other)

Epilepsy is a disruption of the normal electrical activity of the brain causing a seizure. It is a relatively common condition, affecting one in 131 people. No two people experience the same seizure pattern.

If you know you have a person with epilepsy in your care, it is important to ask her or her parent/guardian about the condition and how long her seizures usually last. Epilepsy Action can also provide valuable information (see page 44). The condition has various levels of severity, from minor (absence) seizures to major (tonic clonic) seizures.

Minor seizures

A minor seizure would appear to any onlooker to be a brief loss of concentration.

What to do:

1 Protect the casualty from harm.
2 Ask her to sit down and reassure her, as she may feel confused and disorientated.
3 Give any other first aid as necessary.

Major seizures

A major seizure may last several minutes and involve severe muscular spasms. The casualty may froth at the mouth and have convulsive movements of the body.

What to do:

1 Ensure that anything she might hit herself on, such as furniture, is moved out of the way.
2 Put something soft under her head.
3 Do not try to restrain her.
4 Do not put anything into her mouth.
5 Send for medical help if:
- it is the first seizure
- the seizure is continuing longer than you would expect
- it lasts longer than five minutes
- one seizure is followed closely by another
- she normally only has minor seizures and is now having a major seizure.

6 Put her into the recovery position at the end of a seizure.
7 Continue to monitor her airway, breathing and level of consciousness.

She may sleep for some time following a seizure.

Diabetic emergencies

Diabetes mellitus is a condition in which the body is unable to supply enough insulin to maintain the correct glucose levels. Younger people with diabetes usually treat the condition with injections of insulin. If you know you have someone with diabetes in your care, it is important to ask her or her parent/guardian about the condition and about her regime regarding meals and treatment. Diabetes UK can also provide valuable information (see page 44).

Hypoglycaemia

A person with diabetes is at risk of her blood glucose levels going too low. This is called a hypoglycaemic attack or 'hypo'. It is caused by:
- the dose of insulin being too much for the energy being used
- the person using up more energy than anticipated, eg because of a change in routine or a special or unexpected event
- food intake not being enough for the energy being used
- the person feeling particularly excited
- the weather becoming very hot or very cold.

Symptoms may include:
- shakiness
- sweating
- dizziness
- vagueness.

What to do:

1 Give her some form of sugar immediately, eg a sugar lump, a sweet or a fizzy drink (not diet drinks). If she responds well she should then eat something more substantial, like a sandwich or a bowl of cereal. She will probably be able to recognise the symptoms and be prepared and able to treat herself.
2 If a hypo is left untreated she will eventually lose consciousness. If this happens do not give her anything to eat or drink. Put her into the recovery position (see pages 15–16) and seek medical assistance.

Illness and how it can affect someone with diabetes

Being ill alters the body's functions and can seriously upset the insulin/glucose balance in a person with diabetes. If the person catches a cold or flu she should continue her normal treatment, drink plenty of fluids and, if she is off her food, have small snacks or sugary drinks.

If the person has a stomach upset and sickness or diarrhoea she can become very ill very quickly. In this case seek immediate medical aid.

Most young diabetics monitor their blood glucose levels with the aid of a small machine. This tells them if their diabetes is not controlled and they can regulate their insulin and diet accordingly.

4 OTHER INJURIES AND CONDITIONS

HEAT AND COLD

The body usually maintains an average temperature of 37°C and can naturally cope with normal climate and temperatures. In some conditions this regulation system cannot cope, however, leading to illness.

Heat exhaustion

Heat exhaustion is caused by excessive loss of fluid and salts. This can be prevented by drinking plenty of fluids and avoiding strenuous exercise in excessive heat. A person is more likely to become overheated in a hot, humid environment. This causes:

- headache
- dizziness and confusion
- loss of appetite and nausea
- sweating, with pale, clammy skin
- cramps in the arms, legs or abdomen
- rapid, weakening pulse.

What to do:
1 If possible, move the casualty to a cooler environment.
2 Get him to lie down with his legs elevated.
3 Give him plenty of water or a weak salt-water solution (one teaspoon of salt per litre of water).
4 Seek medical aid.
5 Ensure that everyone else in the group is drinking sufficient fluids.

Heatstroke

Heatstroke is a very serious condition caused by prolonged exposure to heat. It results in serious disruption to the body's temperature-control mechanism. It often follows heat exhaustion but can also be caused by high fever. Symptoms are:

- headache
- dizziness
- discomfort
- restlessness and confusion
- hot, flushed and dry skin
- rapidly lowering levels of response (see page 22)
- a full bounding pulse.

What to do:
1 Move the casualty to a cooler environment.
2 Remove excess clothing.
3 If possible, wrap him in a wet sheet to cool his body.
4 Seek urgent medical aid.

Hypothermia

Hypothermia occurs when the body's temperature has dropped so low that it cannot maintain reflexes (such as shivering) which would return it to the normal range. This is caused by exposure to the cold, combined with insufficient or wet clothing, immersion in water or lack of movement.

Do not assume that this condition is limited to expeditions up mountains. In certain conditions hypothermia may occur on a beach in August! It is important to prevent this by monitoring participants. If you suspect early signs of hypothermia, immediately start to warm up by increasing movement, wrapping and warm drinks.

Symptoms are:
- cold, pale, dry skin
- blue/purple lips
- apathy, irrationality, disorientation and lethargy
- lower levels of consciousness
- slow and shallow breathing
- weakening pulse
- a ceasing of normal reflexes, making the temperature drop even further.

What to do:
1 Protect the casualty from the elements.
2 If possible, replace wet clothing.
3 Place him in warm clothing and a survival/sleeping bag. Keep his head covered.
4 If he is conscious and is able to tolerate them, give him warm drinks.
5 Share body heat and warm air.
6 Try to keep him warm but do not use a direct source of heat such as a hot water bottle.
7 If he becomes unconscious, put him into the recovery position (see pages 15–16).
8 Get urgent medical help.

9 Check other members of the group for the same condition and take preventive measures.

Burns
Burns can be caused by dry heat, friction, radiation (including sunrays), hot liquids, steam and chemicals.

What to do:
1 Immediately cool the skin with cold water for at least ten minutes or until the pain stops.
2 Once cooled, lay a clean, dry, non-fluffy covering, eg a dressing or cling film, over the burn.
3 If possible immediately remove jewellery, watches or other restrictions as the area can swell very quickly.
4 Be prepared for shock to develop and lay the casualty down if you can (see page 19).
5 Do not burst blisters.
6 Leave on any clothing which has stuck to the body.
7 Do not apply anything other than water.
8 Do not apply adhesive dressings.

Seek urgent medical attention if:
- you are in any doubt regarding the burned area
- the burn area is around the mouth or face and affecting the airway
- the burn is severe.

Chemical burns
See also Poisoning (page 26).

Some industrial and domestic chemicals can burn the skin. When going to the aid of someone with chemical burns it is vital to ensure your own safety first. If possible note the name of the chemical.

What to do:

1 Wash the affected area for at least 20 minutes, with the flow of water running away from the casualty. Take care not to splash the chemical onto yourself or the casualty.
2 Chemical burns around the mouth and throat can cause swelling, which can restrict or close the airway, therefore:
● loosen clothing around the neck
● give a conscious casualty sips (never more than this) of cold water
● be prepared to start CPR (see page 16) but remember to protect your mouth from the chemical by using a resuscitation face shield.
3 Get urgent medical help.

Sunburn

See also Heat exhaustion (page 29).

Although sunburn is a common condition, it can be quite serious. It can be prevented by wearing a sun hat and clothes made of natural fibres that cover the whole body, and by using appropriate sun protection cream.

What to do:

1 Move the casualty into a shaded area.
2 Cool the sunburnt area by sponging or showering it with cold water, or get the casualty to soak in a cool bath for at least ten minutes.
3 Seek medical aid if there is extensive blistering or skin damage.

FRACTURES AND SOFT TISSUE INJURIES

Fractures

A fracture is a break or crack in a bone, resulting from some form of force being applied.

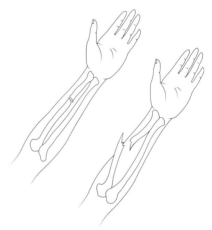

Signs and symptoms may be:
● pain, not necessarily in the area of the fracture as it can travel up or down a nerve (known as 'referred pain')
● lack of mobility or unusual mobility of the limb
● tenderness around the area
● deformity around the fracture area (a lump or bump)
● the sound of a bone breaking
● shock
● bone breaking through the skin
● the casualty may be aware of grating of bones together
● swelling or bruising (usually later).

What to do:

1 If it is a limb, keep it supported, comfortable and still, possibly with the help of a sling (see page 40).
2 Where violent forward or backward bending or twisting (including a fall) has occurred, keep the casualty still, unless his life is threatened, to prevent further injury.
3 Seek medical aid.

Soft tissue injuries (sprains and strains)

A soft tissue injury occurs when a ligament or tendon around a joint has been torn or pulled. This sort of injury can often give similar symptoms to a fracture. If you are in any doubt, treat as a fracture. Remember the mnemonic **RICE** in caring for a soft tissue injury:

R – **R**est the injured part.
I – Apply **I**ce (not directly to the skin) or a cold compress.
C – **C**ompress the injury with padding and a bandage.
E – **E**levate the limb.

MINOR INJURIES
Eye injuries

Injuries to the eye can cause intense pain and should always be treated seriously.

What to do:

1 Give the casualty plenty of reassurance.
2 If possible, flush or irrigate the eye with tepid water.
3 Try not to let the casualty rub the eye.
4 Cover the eye with an eye pad.
5 Seek medical attention.

Foreign bodies in the ears and nose

This is particularly common in young children.

What to do:

1 Reassure the casualty.
2 Keep him quiet and calm.
3 If the foreign body is in the nose, tell him to breathe through his mouth.
4 Seek medical aid.

Minor cuts and grazes

What to do:

1 Wash minor cuts with warm water. (For outdoor activities you can use antiseptic wipes or steripods.)
2 Dry carefully.
3 Apply a plaster, checking whether non-allergic plasters need to be used.
4 Gently rinse grazes to get rid of any particles and then leave to dry naturally.

Nosebleeds

Nosebleeds are fairly common and may be caused by a blow to the nose, picking, sneezing or blowing it. Nosebleeds can lead to considerable loss of blood which, if swallowed, may cause vomiting.

What to do:

1 Apply firm pressure just below the firm part of the nose (you may have to do this for a younger casualty).
2 Get him to sit down and lean forward. If possible, protect his clothing with a cloth or bowl.
3 Try to make sure he does not breathe through his nose, speak,

swallow, cough, spit or sniff.
4 Apply the pressure to his nose for ten minutes. If the bleeding still has not stopped, continue this for a further ten minutes.
5 When the bleeding has stopped, advise him to rest, to avoid exertion and not to pick or blow his nose for a few hours.
6 If the nosebleed persists for longer than 30 minutes, take him to hospital.

If a nosebleed follows a head injury and the blood looks thin and watery this could indicate a very serious condition and urgent medical aid is required.

Tooth loss

What to do:
If a person loses a tooth as a result of an accident, do not wash the tooth.
1 Help the casualty put the tooth back in its socket and keep it in position using a pad, or place the tooth in milk.
2 Get him to a dentist as quickly as possible.

With an older casualty the tooth can be put inside his cheek but must be kept moist.

Splinters

What to do:
1 If the splinter is sticking out of the skin and you are sure of its size, gently try to remove it.

2 If the splinter is large or you are unsure about removing it, seek further medical attention.

Stings (and anaphylaxis)
Insect stings are usually painful as opposed to dangerous.

What to do:
1 Treat initial pain and swelling by cooling the sting with cold water.
2 Remove the sting (if still in) as soon as possible by brushing it away with a plastic card, your nail or something similar.

Occasions when stings can be life threatening:
● multiple stings
● stings in the mouth or throat resulting in swelling which restricts or closes the airway
● a serious allergic reaction (anaphylactic shock, see page 26) to certain insect stings.

If the casualty carries his own medication for dealing with stings, assist him to take his own antidote. It is usually given by injection as a metered dose using an Epipen/ Anapen. Otherwise treat him for shock (see page 18) and seek urgent medical help.

Animal and snake bites
See also Tetanus (page 34).

Animal bites can puncture the skin and carry germs deep into the tissue.

What to do:
1 Reassure the casualty.
2 Control any bleeding.

3 If possible identify the animal, as some pose a greater risk than others.
4 If the casualty has been bitten by a venomous snake, try to keep the bite area below the level of the casualty's heart. Get the casualty to sit quietly.
5 Seek medical aid.

AILMENTS

When caring for young people you will come across a range of minor ailments such as headaches, sore throats, earaches and stomach pains or upsets. How you deal with these will depend upon the situation. At a unit meeting, for example, the casualty may be happy to sit quietly until the end. On a residential event, however, consider carefully what you are told about the condition by the casualty and other adults. He may simply be overtired or the condition could be more serious and require medical attention.

What to do:
1 Reassure the casualty.
2 Try to establish history.
3 Consider how long it will be before a parent/guardian collects the child and whether it might be better to contact them.
4 If you are in any doubt, seek medical advice.

Remember that you may not give any medication unless you have written permission.

Tetanus

If the skin is broken by anything dirty (ie not sterile) check whether the casualty has had a recent tetanus injection. If not, or if you are in any doubt, seek medical attention.

Meningitis

Although it is not a common condition, you should be aware of meningitis. Signs and symptoms are:
- blue lips
- pale and blotching skin
- cold hands and feet
- raised body temperature
- vomiting
- severe headache
- stiff or rigid neck
- feeling very unwell
- photophobia (dislike of light)
- a lowering level of consciousness if untreated
- rash of small purple spots or bruises (when pressed against a glass they do not disappear).

If you have even the smallest suspicion that someone might have meningitis, seek urgent medical advice. Anyone who has been in contact with meningitis will require antibiotic cover.

Contact the Meningitis Trust for more information (see page 44).

SUMMARY

The first person arriving at the scene of an accident or incident should:

- Make the area safe.
- Look out for hidden dangers.
- Reassure the casualty and onlookers.
- Carry out the necessary first aid treatment and arrange for further medical aid as appropriate.
- Inform the parent/guardian of any child that has been unwell or in an accident as soon as possible.
- Carry out notification procedures as stated in the appropriate Association's rules if required (see pages 9–10).
- Record full details of the incident as soon as possible, including:
  - what exactly happened
  - who was involved
  - what you did
  - who you notified.
- Re-stock any first aid equipment you use.

ADDITIONAL TRAINING

For details of organisations that can offer additional training and resources, see pages 43–44. Discuss your needs with your course trainer if you are in doubt. Remember, this course covers only the basic requirements of your Association and for certain activities you will require more training.

INFECTION AND THE FIRST AIDER

Anyone doing first aid needs to be aware of the risk of picking up infection.

Most people are worried about the risk of being infected with HIV, but the principal type of infection that the first aider is exposed to is hepatitis B.

Hepatitis B

A highly contagious and very serious viral infection that affects the liver, often causing jaundice. A carrier may show no signs or symptoms of the virus but it is present in all her body fluids and can remain active outside the body even when the fluids have dried. Immunisation is available for hepatitis B. Contact your doctor/nurse for advice.

HIV

HIV is a virus that attacks the body's immune system, leaving it vulnerable to other infections. The virus is present in all body fluids but dies quickly once outside the body. In first aid situations it can be passed on only by blood-to-blood contact or by contaminated needles breaking the skin. A person carrying the HIV virus may show no signs or symptoms of the infection.

Protecting yourself from infection

The following sensible precautions, most of which are basic hygiene practices and common sense, will go a long way to protect the first aider from contamination:

● Use suitable disposable gloves – if possible you should practise putting gloves on and disposing of them safely.
● Carefully wash your hands after treating a casualty.
● Cover any wounds you have, especially on your hands, with plasters.
● Wash surfaces and other contaminated items after treatment with household bleach diluted 1:10 with water.
● Take care not to prick or cut yourself on any needle or glass.
● Dispose of contaminated waste carefully.
● Use a resuscitation face shield, available from first aid suppliers, when doing mouth-to-mouth resuscitation. Your trainer may show you one and how to use it.

There is no documented evidence of hepatitis B or HIV being passed on during mouth-to-mouth resuscitation.

If you are worried that you may have been infected as a result of undertaking first aid, you should consult your GP or local accident and emergency unit as soon as possible.

For further information on hepatitis B, HIV and AIDS, NHS Direct online has excellent information: www.nhsdirect.nhs.uk .

APPENDIX 2

FIRST AID KITS

The list included is for guidance only. First aiders should think about each event or activity that is taking place, considering the number of participants, the average age of the group and how long the event is going to last.

Used items should be replaced as soon as possible and the kit checked regularly for out-of-date items. Make sure the container and equipment are stored in a suitable place and always kept clean.

No medication should be left in these kits.

Kits should be kept as simple as possible in line with the *Approved Code of Practice Guidance 1997*, amended 2004.

Always remember your training: do not attempt to treat anyone outside of your training guidelines.

The first aid container should be practical for the event or activity – a waterproof material is best – and needs to be marked with either the sign for first aid (white cross on a green circle) or the words 'First aid kit'.

The Health and Safety Executive's *Approved Code of Practice and Guidance 1997* (see Further resources, page 42) gives guidance on workplace first aid kit contents and amounts and is a very useful gauge.

This list is intended as a guide:
- 1 pair disposable non-latex protective gloves
- 20 individually wrapped sterile adhesive dressings
- 2 sterile eye pads
- 6 individually wrapped triangular bandages, preferably sterile
- 6 safety pins
- 6 medium-sized (approximately 12cm x 12cm) individually wrapped sterile unmedicated wound dressings
- 6 large-sized (approximately 18cm x 18cm) individually wrapped sterile unmedicated wound dressings
- guidance leaflet (a leaflet supplied with the kit or that you make yourself which includes brief instructions on emergency treatment).

You might also like to include:
- resuscitation shield
- scissors
- extra gloves
- adhesive tape
- steripods (sealed sachets of normal saline)
- individual wrapped moist cleaning wipes for the first aider's hands.

Remember to have home contact telephone numbers available at all times, plus relevant permission/health forms for the event or activity.

MEDICATION

All medication should be stored in a separate suitable locked container.

Participants should be encouraged to bring any medication they occasionally use, eg travel pills, antihistamines, cold sore medication. These items must be in the original container, be in date and have details for use marked on the label together with the person's name. Details of medication should also be included on Girlguiding UK's health form (G/H), The Scout Association's Camp Holiday Information Form (FS120082) and any other parental consent form used for section meetings and all other activities.

Parents should discuss any conditions and treatment with the Leader or first aider prior to the holiday/camp. The Leader or first aider should be updated with any further details or changes to medication at the start of the holiday/camp, and parents must hand over the medication to the first aider at this point.

General medication

The first aider or Leader may carry a small supply of medicines for the participants' well-being and comfort. You will need parental permission to administer these. Parental permission should be recorded on the appropriate Association's documents.

For Girlguiding UK members, details of these medications should be listed in the marked box on the health form. The Scout Association requires that parental consent be obtained before any medication is given.
Medication may include:

- a form of pain relief such as paracetamol or Calpol (note that aspirin products should not be given to under-16-year-olds)
- sting/bite relief such as Waspeze or Witch doctor
- in travel situations a diarrhoea preparation may be useful, eg Dioralyte, Imodium, Diocalm.

When purchasing any medication, take into consideration the age group of your party and ask the pharmacist for advice.

You may prefer not to carry any medication but you should discuss this with your group's parents/guardians.

Note on antiseptic cream
The use of antiseptic cream is not encouraged at any time. Research has shown that antiseptic creams delay healing.

It is advised that wounds are kept clean with warm water and kept covered, especially in situations where it is difficult to maintain cleanliness, such as at camp.

APPENDIX **3**

ELEVATION AND ARM SLING

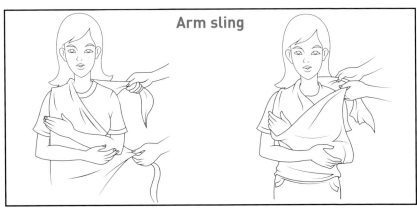

Arm sling

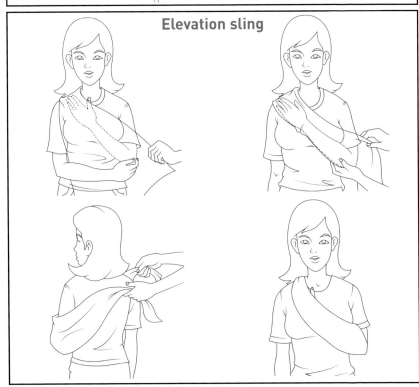

Elevation sling

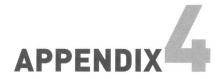
APPENDIX 4

CHAIN OF SURVIVAL

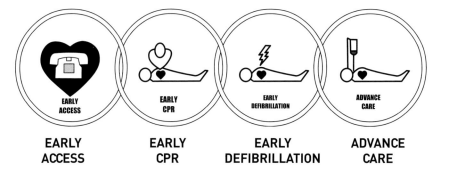

| EARLY ACCESS | EARLY CPR | EARLY DEFIBRILLATION | ADVANCE CARE |

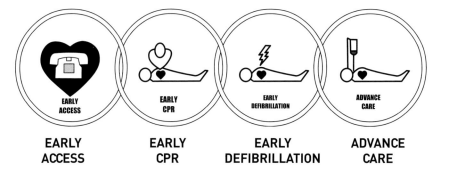

EARLY ACCESS   **EARLY CPR**   **EARLY DEFIBRILLATION**   **ADVANCE CARE**

FURTHER RESOURCES

First Aid
First Aid Manual, St Andrews Ambulance, St. John Ambulance and the British Red Cross, Dorling Kindersley, ISBN 0 75133 704 8
First Aid at Work: The Health and Safety (First Aid) Regulations 1981. Approved Code of Practice and Guidance L74, HSE Books 1997, ISBN 0 71761 050 0

Girlguiding UK publications
Girlguiding UK Trading Service order codes in brackets
The Guiding Manual (6455)
What you need to know about safety (6057)
Starting Rainbows/Brownies/Guides: Notes for parents and guardians (6164/6808/6519)
Training opportunities: Catering and health and first aid schemes (6480)
Rainbow overnights (6694) / *Going away with Brownies* (6695) / *Going away with Guides* (6696) / *Going away with the Senior Section* (6697)
Safe From Harm: Good practice for adults in guiding (available from Commissioners and Country/Region offices, and in the Leadership Qualification pack (6623))

Scout Association publications
The Scout Association Information Centre codes in brackets
Accidents: Leaders'/Commissioners' Guide to Reporting (FS120079)
First Aid Kits and Accident Books (FS140048)
Home Contacts (FS120078)
Camp Holiday Information Form (FS120082)
Policy, Organisation and Rules (LT435000)
Special Needs Factsheets: Epilepsy (FS250011), *Asthma* (FS250018), *Diabetes* (FS250009), *Allergies* (FS250051), *Appropriate Medical Care* (FS322101)
What Price Accidents? (FS320001)
Young People First (YC)
Risk Assessments (FS120000)
First Response: Definitions and Equivalents (FS310547)

First aiders and other readers should always ensure that they are using the most recent edition of any of these publications. During the lifespan of this publication new resources may be published by Girlguiding UK and The Scout Association or other publishers: keeping up to date with current practice and appropriate resources is the responsibility of individuals.

APPENDIX 6

USEFUL ADDRESSES
Girlguiding UK
GIRLGUIDING UK (CHQ)
17–19 Buckingham Palace Road
London SW1W 0PT
Tel: 020 7834 6242
Fax: 020 7828 8317
Email: chq@girlguiding.org.uk
Website: www.girlguiding.org.uk

GIRLGUIDING UK TRADING SERVICE
Atlantic Street
Broadheath
Altrincham
Cheshire WA14 5EQ
Tel: 0161 941 2237
Fax: 0161 941 6326

INSURANCE
AON Girlguiding UK Insurance Service
PO Box 410
Redhill
RH1 1AW
Tel: 0870 240 3706
Email: girlguiding@ars.aon.co.uk

The Scout Association
For first aid enquiries:
THE ADULT TRAINING OFFICE
The Scout Association
Gilwell Park
Bury Road
Chingford E4 7QW
Tel: 0845 300 1818
Email: adult.support@scout.org.uk

For accident reporting:
THE INFORMATION CENTRE
The Scout Association
Gilwell Park
Bury Road
Chingford E4 7QW
Tel: 0845 300 1818
Email: info.centre@scout.org.uk

For insurance enquiries:
SCOUT INSURANCE SERVICES LTD
Lancing Business Park
Lancing
West Sussex BN15 8UG
Tel: 01903 768524
Email: scouts@siscolan.co.uk

Health and first aid organisations
THE ANAPHYLAXIS CAMPAIGN
Tel: 01252 542029
Email: info@anaphylaxis.org.uk
Website: www.anaphylaxis.org.uk

ASTHMA UK
Tel: 08457 01 02 03
Website: www.asthma.org.uk

THE BRITISH HEART FOUNDATION
Heartstart UK
14 Fitzhardinge Street
London W1H 6DH
Tel: 020 7935 0185
Email: heartstart@bhf.org.uk
Website: www.bhf.org.uk

BRITISH RED CROSS
UK Office
44 Moorfields
London EC2Y 9AL
Tel: 0870 170 7000
Email: firstaid@redcross.org.uk
Website: www.redcross.org.uk/firstaid

DIABETES UK
Tel: 020 7424 1000
Email: info@diabetes.org.uk
Website: www.diabetes.org.uk

EPILEPSY ACTION
Tel: 0113 210 8800
Email: epilepsy@epilepsy.org.uk
Website: www.epilepsy.org.uk

HEALTH AND SAFETY EXECUTIVE
HSE Information Centre
Broad Lane
Sheffield S3 7HQ
Tel: 0845 345 0055
Website: www.hse.gov.uk

MENINGITIS TRUST HEAD OFFICE
Fern House
Bath Road
Stroud GL5 3TJ
Tel: 01453 768000
24-hour nurse led helpline:
0800 028 18 28
Email: info@meningitis-trust.org
Website: www.meningitis-trust.org

NHS DIRECT
Tel: 0845 4647
Website: www.nhsdirect.nhs.uk

RESUSCITATION COUNCIL (UK)
5th floor
Tavistock House North
Tavistock Square
London WC1H 9HR
Tel: 020 7388 4678
Email: enquiries@resus.org.uk
Website: www.resus.org.uk

ST. ANDREW'S AMBULANCE ASSOCIATION
St. Andrew's House
48 Milton Street
Glasgow G4 0HR
Tel: 0141 332 4031
Email: firstaid@staaa.org.uk
Website: www.firstaid.org.uk

ST. JOHN AMBULANCE ASSOCIATION
National Headquarters
27 St John's Lane
London EC1M 4BU
Tel: 08700 10 49 50
Website: www.sja.org.uk

Further training

Please note that 1st Response is not a qualification. Details of assessed qualifications can be sought from any of the external organisations listed above.

1ST RESPONSE
Attendance certificate

THIS IS TO CERTIFY THAT

....

HAS COMPLETED THE
1ST RESPONSE COURSE

DATE ....

COURSE TUTOR ....

RENEWED ....

DATE ....

RENEWED ....

DATE ....

Renewable every three years